How Your Favorite Meal Could be Killing You Slowly

Health Learning Series

Colvin Nyakundi

Mendon Cottage Books

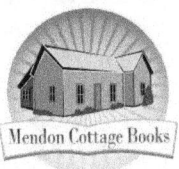 

JD-Biz Publishing

Our books are available at
1. Amazon.com
2. Barnes and Noble
3. Itunes
4. Kobo
5. Smashwords
6. Google Play Books

Table of Contents

Introduction 4

Meals Associated With Common Chronic Diseases............................5

Popular Natural and Healthy Meals 10

Dangerous Ingredients to Look Out For 13

What You Must Know About Alcoholic Drinks..............................15

Signs That Your Health Is Deteriorating.............................18

How to live a healthy lifestyle................................21

Conclusion..24

Author Bio..25

Publisher..35

Introduction

According to American Diabetes Association, there are about 25.8 million diabetic Americans as of 2013. Each year about 1.9 million more Americans are diagnosed with diabetes. Millions of Americans also live with other chronic and acute diseases including cancer, rheumatoid arthritis and coronary artery disease. Whereas some of these medical conditions can be treated or controlled, there are those that are simply incurable. Even those that can be treated will have a huge impact on your financial status especially if you don't have sufficient medical insurance cover. It is also possible that such diseases may affect your general health and body immune system. With all these facts, it is up to you to take measures to avoid them.

Throughout the world, countless scientific research projects have been commissioned in order to unravel the causes and cures to chronic and acute diseases. Even though there is no known common cause of all these diseases, scientists generally agree that some meals and lifestyles increase the probability of acquiring such diseases. This means that you must always be very careful about what you frequently eat or drink.

Some meals and drinks have positive health benefits but may negatively affect your health if taken in excessive amounts. It is therefore your responsibility to eat or drink in moderation. Your general lifestyle could also affect your health and lead to conditions such as obesity.

With the book 'How Your Favorite Meal Could Be Killing You Slowly' you'll have an insight into the meals that may negatively affect your health. By reading this book, you'll also learn the ingredients to avoid when buying convenience meals. If you're interested in natural, healthy meals, all you need to do is read this book and you'll know how to go about it.

Live a long and healthy lifestyle by reading the book: How Your Favorite Meal Could Be Killing You Slowly!!!

Meals Associated With Common Chronic Diseases

Due to their busy lifestyles, more and more Americans are going for convenience foods instead of preparing meals at their home. The yummy nature of these convenience meals is also part of the reason as to why they are so popular in most American homes. However, do you known that these meals could be having a negative impact on your health.

Most of these meals contain preservatives and other chemicals that aren't poisonous when taken in small quantities but negatively affect your health when consumed over a long period of time. In some cases, accumulation of such chemicals in the human body may be fatal. Apart from avoiding convenience meals it is also important that you avoid meals with high fat content as they increase the probability of a stroke or high blood pressure. You should therefore be very careful about what you cook if you decide to prepare your own meals. Here are some of the meals that may be killing you slowly by negatively affecting your health:

- A lot of bacon

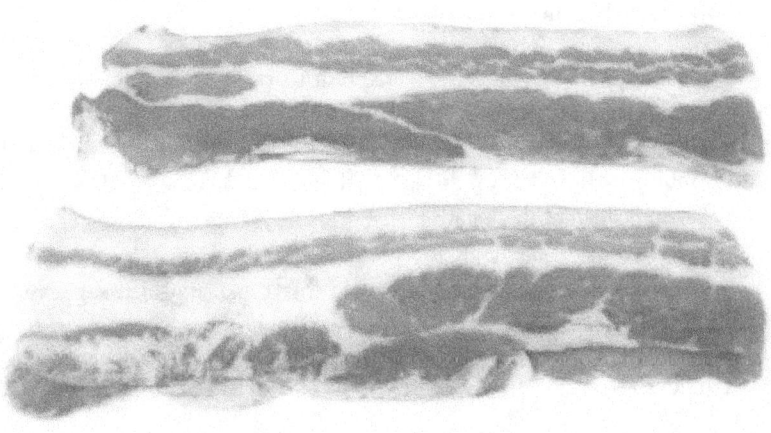

Are you so fond of bacon that you can't stay the whole day without tasting some? If that is the case, then you need to change your lifestyle or else risk a stroke. According to nutrition experts around the world, heavy consumption of bacon significantly increases chances of a stroke in adults. A stroke on the other hand may lead to paralysis or even death. If you don't want to spend the rest of your life bedridden or on a wheelchair, then you need to consider cutting down on your intake of bacon.

- Canned tomato sauce

Most American families rarely miss canned tomato sauce in their homes due to its tastiness and affordability. What most of them don't know is that the high sugar levels in canned tomato sauce could have a negative impact on their health. It is therefore important that you stop or reduce the amount of canned tomato sauce you consume so as to live a healthy lifestyle. If possible canned tomato sauce should be replaced with other natural products as discussed in another chapter in this book.

- Convenience deep-fried foods

You need to think twice before buying one of your favorite convenience deep-fried foods such as chicken, donuts or French fries. The high fat content in most of these meals may clog veins and thus lead to high blood pressure. Such meals also lead to obesity. According to findings from several scientific researches, convenience deep-fried meals may also lead to certain types of cancers.

- Popular carbonated soft drinks

It is on record that one of the most popular soft drink companies in the world is planning to drop a major ingredient in its soft drinks as a result of it being associated with certain types of cancers. This is a clear indicator that you should stop over-drinking carbonated soft drinks. There are several other healthy drinks that can be taken instead of these carbonated drinks. Apart from causing cancer, the high acid levels in most of the popular carbonated soft drinks may lead to tooth decay. The preservatives included in carbonated soft drinks may also negatively affect your health when consumed over a long period of time.

- Hotdogs

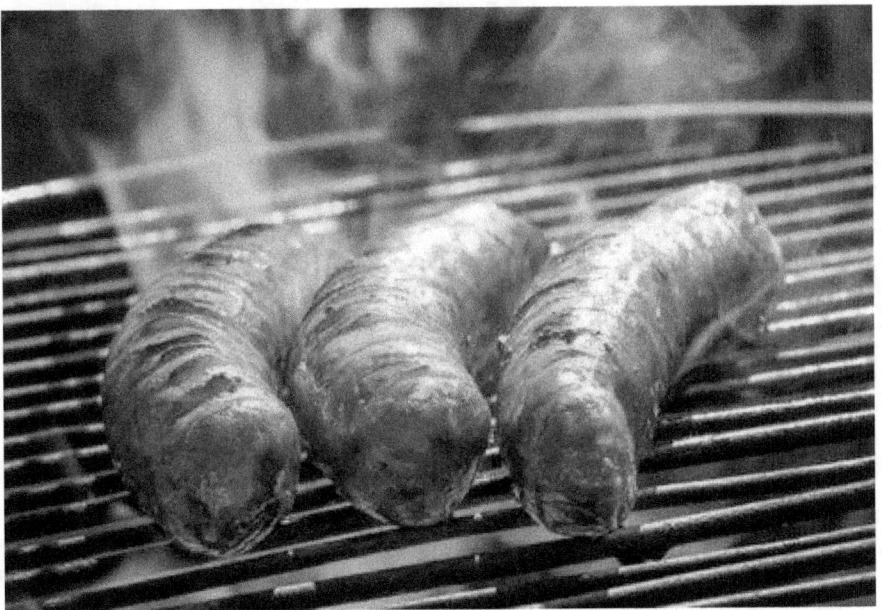

Hotdogs are some of the most popular fast foods among youths and middle age Americans. Actually some people eat hotdogs several times a day due to its sweet taste and convenience. If hotdogs are some of your favorite snacks, then you need to consider going for something else because you are risking contracting colorectal cancer (Colorectal cancer is cancer that affects the colon and rectum). According to scientists, hotdogs increase the probability of acquiring colorectal cancer by about 21%.

- Potato chips

The high fat content in potato chips makes you prone to heart attacks and high blood pressure. Potato chips are also associated with certain types of cancers. It is therefore very important that you avoid potato chips as much as possible.

- Ready meat

Have you ever wondered why packaged meat takes longer to go bad? Well, they contain several preservatives that may just lead to your health problems. Some preservatives are associated with certain types of cancers and also affect your body hormones and immune system. It is therefore your responsibility to avoid ready meat. Rather than going for ready meat, you should just buy meat from the local butcher even if it will go bad sooner.

- Whole milk

You need to think twice before feeding your child whole milk. Scientific analyses of whole milk show that it contains high levels of bovine growth hormone. These hormone leads to obesity in children if consumed in excessive quantities. You should therefore limit the amount of whole milk taken by your child so that he/she doesn't become one of those obese and unhealthy kids. Keep in mind that obesity generally leads to poor immune system in the child's body.

- Yogurt

Yogurt is a favorite soft drink especially among children. However, this sweet drink should be discouraged due to the high amounts of fructose corn syrup added as a sweetener. When processing yogurt, preservatives are also added so as to increase its shelf life. Some of these preservatives are poisonous if consumed over a long period of time. Health problems associated with excessive intake of yogurt includes obesity in children.

- Ice cream

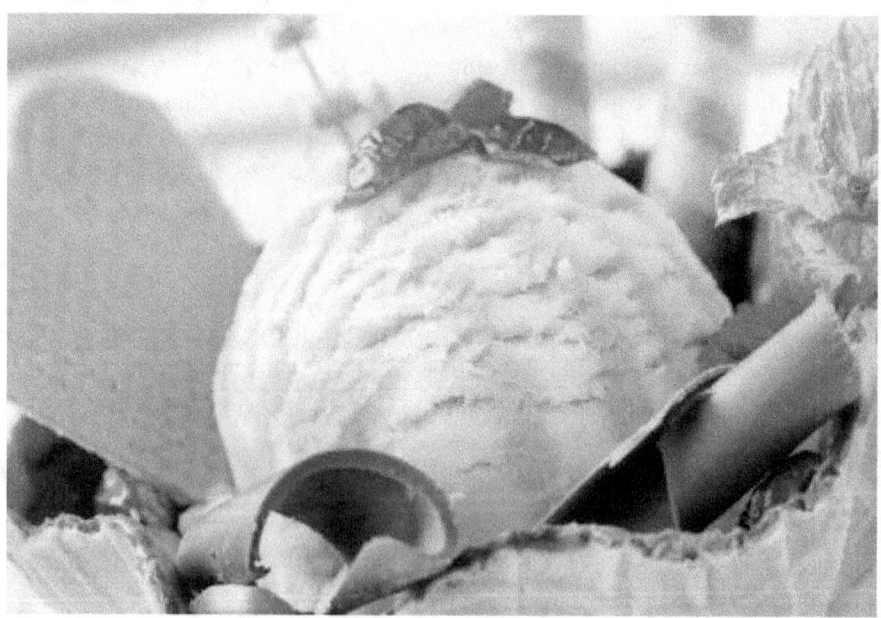

The sweet nature of ice cream makes most people to buy more and more of it every day. You should however limit your consumption of ice cream as it contains high levels of cholesterol. Keep in mind that cholesterol increases chances of contracting high blood pressure among many other ailments.

- Chocolate

You need to reconsider your preferences if you're fond of eating chocolate. Apart from the fact that the high sugar content can lead to tooth decay, chocolates may also contain dangerous/unhealthy ingredients.

- Margarine

For most people, margarine is the best and cheapest alternative to butter. Some people can't even imagine of eating bread without margarine. However, do you know that margarine contains high cholesterol levels even if it is made from natural products? High cholesterol levels clog blood vessels reducing their diameter and hence leading to high blood pressure. Excessive consumption of margarine is also associated with obesity and strokes. You must therefore recognize the importance of reducing margarine consumption if you're interested in living a healthy lifestyle.

- Snacks with enriched wheat flour

Enriched wheat flour is one of the ingredients that you should try to avoid when buying snacks. Nutritionists generally agree that enriched wheat flour may weaken your body and compromise your immune system.

- Excessive consumption of eggs

Eggs are generally considered to be natural and healthy meals as long as they're not consumed excessively. Apart from the protein in eggs which helps in growth and replacement of dead body cells, they also contain fat and cholesterol that may lead to high blood pressure. It is therefore very important that you reduce your daily consumption of eggs. If you can't avoid cutting down on your egg consumption, then you have to increase the number of hours you spend exercising.

Popular Natural and Healthy Meals

There are so many natural and healthy meals that will positively affect your health. Apart from increasing your body immune system, these meals can help you avoid obesity and some types of cancers. Nutrition experts around the world have a consensus that these meals may increase your lifespan and reduce the probability of falling ill. The best thing about most of these natural and healthy meals is that they are readily and cheaply available in most parts of the world. Here are some of the things that you can eat so as to live a healthy and long lasting life:

- Water

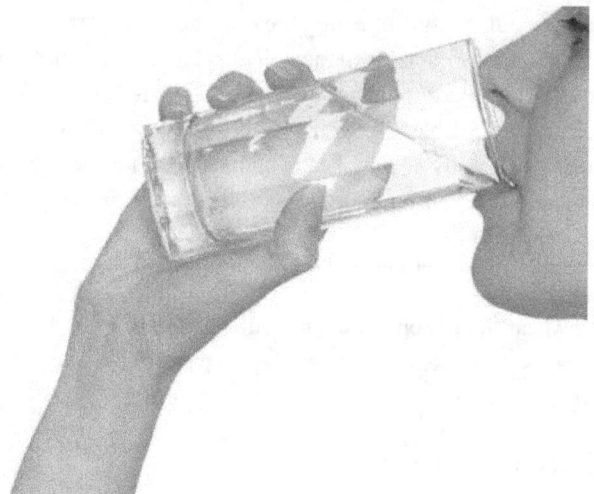

There is a lot of debate worldwide about whether water should be categorized as a meal or just a drink. In spite of that, it is generally accepted to be the best drink for anybody who is feeling thirsty. Rather than buying your favorite soda, you should consider drinking water due to its positive impact on your health and immune system. As a matter of fact, more than three quarters of human body cells are made of water. More than 70% of the world's surface is also filled with water. One more advantage of consuming water is that it is not known to cause any negative effect on a human being's health.

- Honey

Rather than buying artificial sweeteners you should consider going for honey. This sweet, yellow product is known to have several health benefits as it is not taken through any form of industrial processing. Honey also doesn't need any preservatives and therefore you can rest assured it is as natural as possible.

- Natural tomatoes instead of canned tomatoes

When processing tomatoes, manufacturers normally add sweeteners, preservatives and food colors. Some of the chemicals used in the manufacture of these ingredients may harm you if consumed over prolonged periods of time. It is therefore important that you eat unprocessed tomatoes directly from the farm instead of going for the canned ones.

- Natural pepper instead of processed pepper

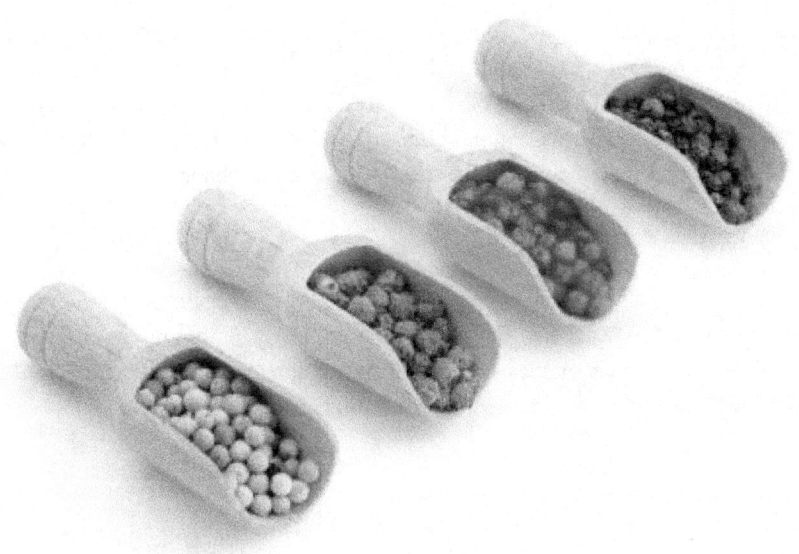

Even though you may not know, processing pepper involves several stages through which numerous additives and preservatives are added. In some countries, manufacturers prefer using the cheap and easily available chemicals synthesized in the lab instead of natural pepper as the raw material. Some of these chemicals are dangerous if consumed continuously for a long time. If you are one of those people who cannot eat any meal without the tingling sensation of pepper, then you need to consider going for fresh pepper straight from the farm.

- Avocado and olive oil instead of margarine

Unlike margarine, avocados and olive oils are natural and contain lower amounts of cholesterol. This means that by simply consuming avocado and olive oil you can significantly reduce chances of a stroke or high blood pressure. However, you need to note that excessive consumption of these natural products may also negatively affect you as they have some cholesterol.

- Blended mango juice instead of industrial juices

Some companies claim that their products are natural and healthy but it is a fact that preservatives have to be included. So, why not just buy mangoes from your local grocer and blend your own juice? You'll be avoiding artificial sweeteners, preservatives and other ingredients that may negatively affect your health.

- Milk

Even though whole milk contains high levels of bovine growth hormone, milk generally consists of calcium and phosphorous that strengthens bones and thus reducing the risk of malformation in children. By giving your child correct amounts of milk you can help them avoid rickets and several other abnormalities.

- Vegetables

Vegetables and meals with high fiber content are known to improve the human digestive system. You can therefore boost your health by simply increasing your daily consumption of vegetables such as spinach. Remember that these vegetables also contain other important nutrients in addition to their fiber content.

- Carrots

Scientific research indicates that carrots contain nutrients that help improve eyesight. If you've been having problems with your eyes, maybe you need to consider increasing your intake of carrots. However, you should note that it may take long for you to notice the effect of eating carrots. It is therefore your responsibility to visit your doctor in case you are having problems with your eyesight.

Other natural, tasty and healthy farm products that you should consider adding to your favorite meals include lemons, bananas, apples, strawberry, peaches, fig, pineapple and garlic. You should consider growing some of these farm products in your backyard since they generally grow in almost all environmental conditions. They also require minimal care and they'll save you the money that could have been spent at the local grocer.

Dangerous Ingredients to Look Out For

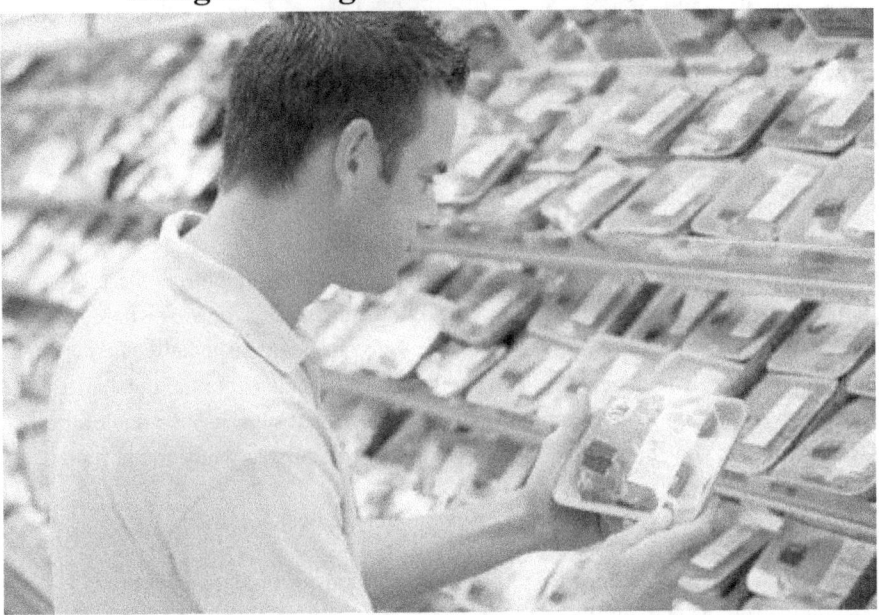

You shouldn't be surprised to hear that most people never bother to check the labeling in their favorite processed/fast foods before purchasing them. In spite of this, the Food and Drug Administration (FDA) mandates manufacturers to properly label their products and highlight all the ingredients in the meal. It is therefore your responsibility to check the label and determine the ingredient included in your favorite meal. You should always keep in mind that some of these ingredients are known to increase the probability of acquiring certain types of cancers. Some people are allergic to some ingredients and may have to be admitted in hospital after consuming the ingredient they're allergic to. Some of the ingredients you should be cautious about include the following:

- Brominated Vegetable Oil (BVO)

Brominated vegetable oil is one of the most preferred preservatives among manufacturers. However, this industrial chemical is dangerous and may lead to several health problems if consumed in large amounts. You should therefore be on the lookout for this preservative whenever buying any ready-for-consumption meal.

- Caramel coloring

Some companies would do anything to make sure that they attract as many people as possible. They therefore include attractive food colors that make their products look yummy. This is one of the reasons as to why caramel coloring is quite popular in spite of its negative effects when consumed in large quantities. Before you pay for any meal, make sure that this food color is not included in the ingredients.

- Artificial sweeteners

After several stages of processing and addition of preservatives, ready-to-eat meals may not be as tasty as many people would want. Most manufacturers therefore opt to include artificial sweeteners so as to make the convenience meals tastier. Some of these sweeteners may have a negative impact on your health especially if consumed in high amounts. Sweeteners that you should avoid include neotame, saccharin, sucralose, acesulfame potassium and aspartame. Refined sugar is also one of the sweeteners that you should try to avoid whenever purchasing ready-made foods.

- Hydrolyzed vegetable proteins and autolyzed yeast extract

When consumed in high doses over prolonged periods of time, hydrolyzed vegetable proteins and autolyzed yeast extract may make you prone to certain diseases. You should therefore be always on the lookout for these ingredients and try to avoid them as much as possible.

Other ingredients that are associated with common diseases include brown sugar, corn syrup, dextrin, dextrose, high fructose corn syrup, malto-dextrin, molasses, monosodium glutamate and partially hydrogenated oil.

So, the next time you're in your local department store, don't just buy any packaged meal. You should first take a look at the label so as to ascertain the ingredients in the meal. Keep in mind that manufacturers never tell you their ingredients when marketing their products. They just try to convince you to buy their products blindly.

What You Must Know About Alcoholic Drinks

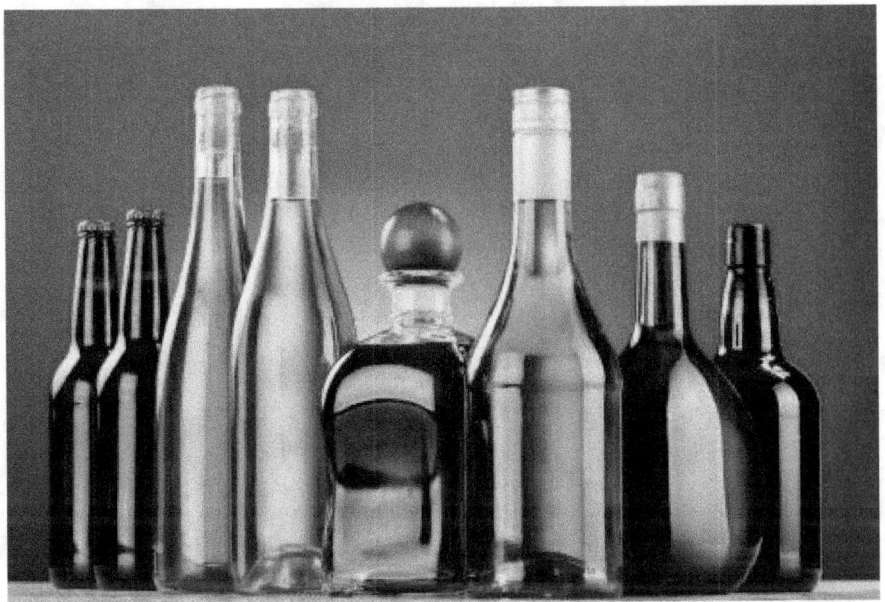

Alcohol is a drink that has been part of human civilization for thousands of years. This drink is quite popular in most parts of the world with the exception of majority Muslim countries. Scientifically, alcohol can be defined as a drink with 3 to 40% ethanol. Depending on the processing method or procedure, alcoholic drinks can be categorized as wines, spirits or beer.

When drunk in moderation, alcoholic drinks have a positive impact on a human's health. However, if over-consumed alcohol has countless negative effects and may lead to premature death. For an adult to be categorized as a moderate drinker they need to consume a maximum of 2 bottles of beer per day for men and 1 bottle of beer per day for women. Moderate drinkers stand to benefit from the following health advantages of alcohol:

- Reduced risk of cardiovascular disease

Scientific researches indicate that drinking alcohol in moderation helps reduce the risk of contracting cardiovascular disease. Cardiovascular diseases are diseases affecting the human heart or blood vessels.

- Prevent common cold

Even though common cold is not fatal and generally heals after some time even without medication, it makes the affected individual very uncomfortable. It may also affect your performance and probably force you to stay indoors or away from work for a couple of days. By drinking alcohol in moderation, you can reduce the probability of contracting common cold.

- Increase your libido

Are you having problems in lovemaking? Studies indicate that people who consume alcohol have a higher libido when compared to those who don't drink. You can therefore boost your libido by taking a few bottles of beer before going to bed. However, you still need to visit your doctor so as to get proper advice on how to improve your libido without consuming alcohol.

- Lowers chances of getting diabetes

Diabetes is a disease characterized by abnormally high glucose levels in the blood stream. Common symptoms of diabetes include frequent urination and persistent thirst. Drinking the recommended amounts of alcohol reduces chances of acquiring diabetes.

- Temporary reduction in pain

Alcohol can temporarily reduce pain from an injury because of its effect on the nervous system. However alcohol should not be construed for drugs administered by qualified medical practitioners. This means that you should not just go drinking alcohol whenever you feel pain.

In spite of the many advantages of drinking alcohol, alcoholism can have a huge negative impact on your health and general lifestyle. Some of the disadvantages of excessive consumption of alcohol include the following:

- cirrhosis

Cirrhosis is a chronic disease in which the normal functioning of the liver is affected. Scientists generally agree that liver cirrhosis is caused by excessive consumption of alcohol. In some cases, liver cirrhosis may lead to other ailments or even death. If you're keen on avoiding cirrhosis, then you have to cut down on your consumption of alcohol.

- May lead to addiction

One of the major disadvantages of excessive consumption of alcohol is that it may lead to addiction. Some people are so much addicted to alcohol that they can't concentrate on anything or do something useful without taking some alcohol. This kind of dependence on alcohol can negatively affect your performance while at work or even at home.

- Impaired judgment

Impaired judgment is a situation in which one cannot distinguish something just the way it is. When your judgment is impaired, everything looks distorted and it is quite difficult to make correct decisions or approximations. Consumption of excessive amounts of alcohol impairs your judgment. It is therefore advisable that you don't drink and/or drive or operate machinery. Remember that it is your life at stake here.

- May lead to anemia

Anemia is a medical condition characterized by low levels of red blood cells in the blood stream. Red blood cells carry oxygen from the lungs to various parts of the body. With insufficient red blood cells, you will be generally weak and body organs may start developing problems. Excessive consumption of alcohol may lead to anemia and hence should be avoided as much as possible.

If not drunk in moderation alcohol may lead to other conditions such as depression, seizures and dementia. Alcohol abuse may also affect your social life and general behavior.

Signs That Your Health Is Deteriorating

If diagnosed early, some diseases such as cancer may be completely cured or controlled. Cancer is the abnormal growth of body cells as a result of uncontrolled cell division. The disease is characterized by malignant growth or tumor(s) that may spread to other parts of the body through blood vessels or the lymphatic system. If not detected early enough, it is quite difficult to treat cancer and leads to death within just a few months or years. It is therefore quite important for you to be on the lookout for symptoms of this and all other diseases. Some of the following symptoms could indicate that your health is deteriorating.

- Obesity

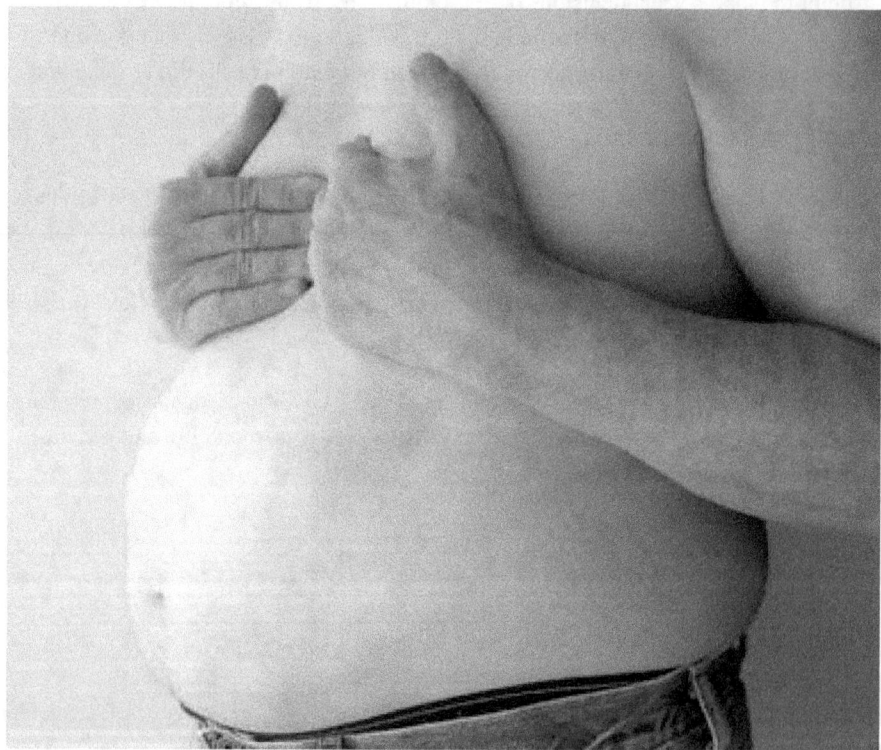

Have you noticed that your weight has been increasing at an abnormal rate in the past few weeks or months? This could indicate that you've been consuming so much fat which is affecting your health. You therefore need to change your diet or visit your doctor for advice on how to live a healthy lifestyle.

- Tooth decay

Tooth decay can indicate that you've been drinking a lot of soda of late. Since sodas have other chemicals that negatively affect your health, you need to reduce your consumption of these carbonated beverages. Over-consumption of sugar could also lead to tooth decay.

- Breathing problems

Abnormal/infected lungs could lead to breathing problems even to those people who rarely fall ill. You should therefore be worried if you've been having breathing problems in the recent past.

- Ageing faster than your age-mates

One of the symptoms of deteriorating health is that you are likely to appear much older than your actual age. This means that you should consult your doctor immediately if wrinkles start appearing on your face at an early age than your age-mates.

- Changes in your skin and hair

Something could be wrong with your health if your skin and hair change color suddenly and rapidly even without the application of any skin products. You therefore need to visit a doctor immediately if you noticed abnormal changes to your skin and hair.

- Behavioral issues in children

Deteriorating health in children could lead to sudden changes in behavior and mood swings. You should therefore visit your pediatrician, if your child's behavior changes abruptly.

- Lack of concentration in whatever you're doing

There is something wrong with your health if you're not concentrating on anything of late. However, you should not be worried if you've been taking medication that might have affected your concentration level.

- Feeling tired always

Fatigue even when you've not done any physical task could be an indication that your health is degenerating. You should therefore visit your doctor as soon as you start experiencing this symptom.

- Chronic migraines

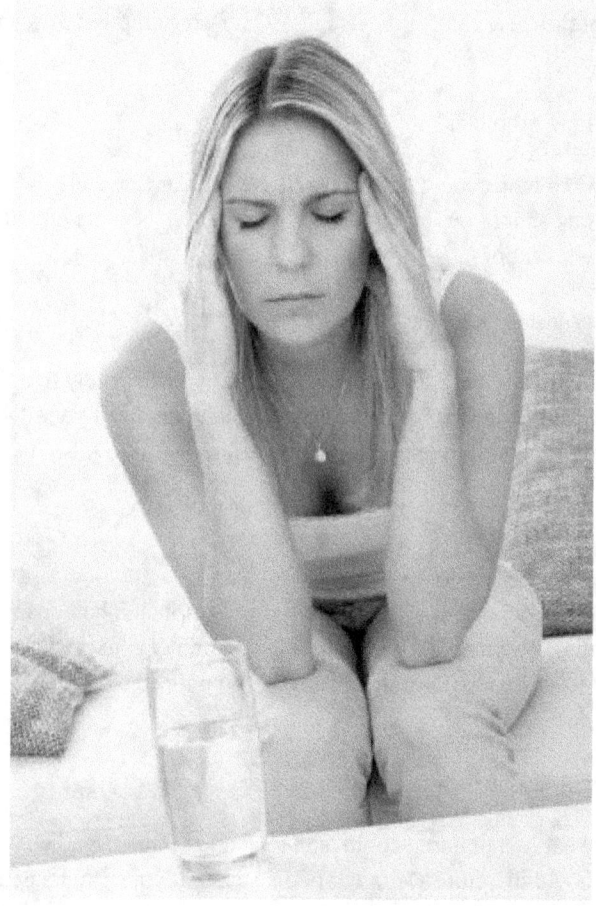

If you've been experiencing severe and persistent headaches even after taking painkillers, then your health could be disintegrating slowly. It is therefore up to you to visit your doctor and find out what is causing the chronic headaches.

- Liver and kidney problems

The liver and kidney are some of the most important organs in the human body. Without these vital organs, the human body cannot work properly and you may die unless you seek immediate medical attention. The kidney is used to filter unwanted particles in the blood stream. Signs of kidney failure include swelling of body parts including the legs and face.

How to live a healthy lifestyle

Lifestyle or 'modus Vivendi' can be defined as the manner of living that reflects your values and attitude towards other people and everything near you. It is irrefutable that lifestyle is one of the main determinants of the lifespan in a given population. You can therefore significantly reduce chances of dying young by simply living a healthy lifestyle. Here are some of the things that you should do if you're keen on living a healthy lifestyle:

- Regular exercises

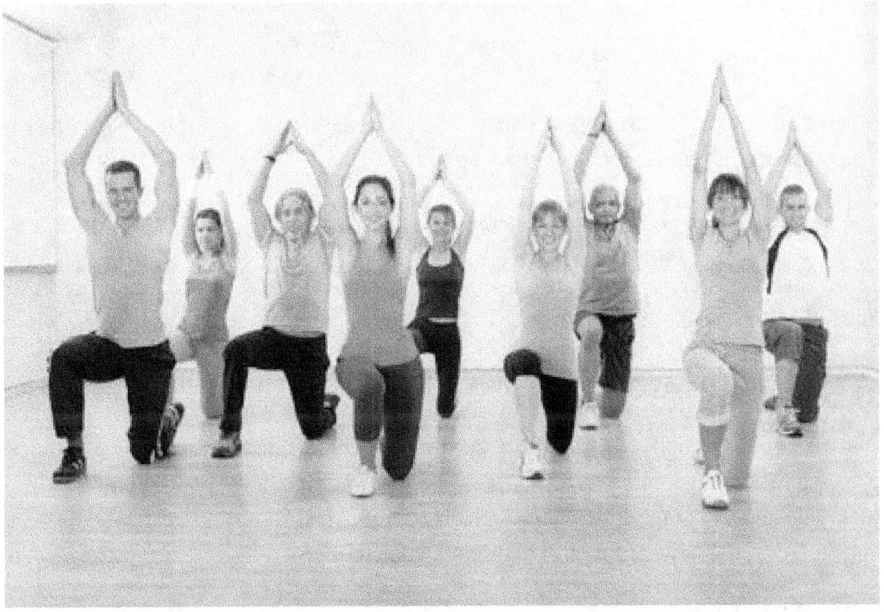

Apart from helping 'burn' the excess fat in your body, regular exercises strengthen bones and body tissues. Frequent exercises have also been linked to improved immune system in human beings. You should therefore include exercises in your daily routine so as to make sure that you live a healthy lifestyle. If possible, you can visit a physical education (PE) expert to help you determine the kind of exercises to include in your routine.

- Healthy and balanced diet

As discussed earlier, some meals make you susceptible to certain types of chronic and/or acute diseases. You must therefore ensure that you always eat meals with no negative effects on your health. It is also important that you consume balanced diet so as to improve your general health and immune system.

- Be hygienic

By being hygienic, you can avoid waterborne diseases among many other ailments. It is therefore your responsibility to be as clean as possible.

- Exposure to toxic chemicals

Avoid exposure to toxic chemicals whenever at home or work. If you're dealing with dangerous chemicals, make sure that you use protective gear.

- Regular medical checkups

Some diseases may be treated if detected/diagnosed early enough. This means that you must go for regular medical checkups.

- Cut down your intake of alcoholic drinks

Just as discussed early on in this book, you must avoid excessive consumption of alcohol.

- Avoid smoking

Apart from the addictive nature of tobacco in cigarettes, there are so many health problems associated with smoking. For instance, smoking makes you prone to tuberculosis and certain types of cancers. You must therefore stake responsibility and stop or reduce the number of cigarettes you smoke.

- Enough sleep

Scientists across the world generally agree that enough sleep is one of the vital ingredients in a healthy lifestyle. Enough sleep helps the human brain rest and recoup the energy required to stay awake the following day. You should therefore get enough sleep each day as per the recommended number of hours.

- Avoid depression and stress

Being depressed and stressed for a long period of time could have a negative impact on your health. For instance, researchers link ulcers in adults to stress. You should therefore avoid factors or people that stress you.

Conclusion

Your health is one of the things that you should never take for granted for as long as you're alive. With degenerating health, you can't be able to perform optimally whenever at work or home. You're also likely to have a bad social life if you're not careful about your health. You must take responsibility and change your lifestyle and the meals you take since they significantly affect your health.

Apart from avoiding meals with poisonous/dangerous ingredients, it is important that you avoid expired meals and also those with ingredients you're allergic to. Keep in mind that most of these dangerous ingredients won't affect you when consumed in small amounts but affect your general health over long periods of time. Just because your favorite fast food is certified by the Food and Drug Administration (FDA) doesn't mean that it won't affect your health in the long run.

Checking the labels in convenience meals is one of the measures you can take so as to make sure that you consume meals with no poisonous ingredients. You must also make sure that you only buy convenience meals from credible companies. Some time back unsuspecting beef lovers in Europe were eating horse meat while thinking it is beef. The company responsible for this mess had duped them into believing that they were eating beef.

It is very unfortunate that some people know the importance of eating healthy meals but choose to ignore and continue eating unhealthy meals. Living a healthy lifestyle is also very important if you're a parent because your children could be trying to emulate you. For instance, your children can become alcoholics if you're also an alcoholic. Your eating habits are also likely to be replicated to those closest to you.

Author Bio

Colvin Tonya Nyakundi

Colvin Tonya Nyakundi is a professional freelance writer and co-author of 'How Your Favorite Meal Could Be Killing You Slowly.' Apart from that book, he has a portfolio of several other publications accumulated in the more than two years that he has been freelancing through www.odesk.com.

In addition to his interest in' healthy lifestyle' publications he has authored several personal relationships, survival, travel and holiday guides, and real estate publications. Other books that he has co-authored include 'How to Improve Your Communication Skills,' 'Construction Guide for New Investors in Real Estate,' 'How to Make Your Backyard a Magnificent Venue for Hosting Events', 'How to Identify the Perfect Holiday Destination' and How to Prepare and Survive in a Foreign Country.' You can get in touch with him through his official Facebook account, tonyanc@facebook.com.

Check out some of the other JD-Biz Publishing books

Gardening Series on Amazon

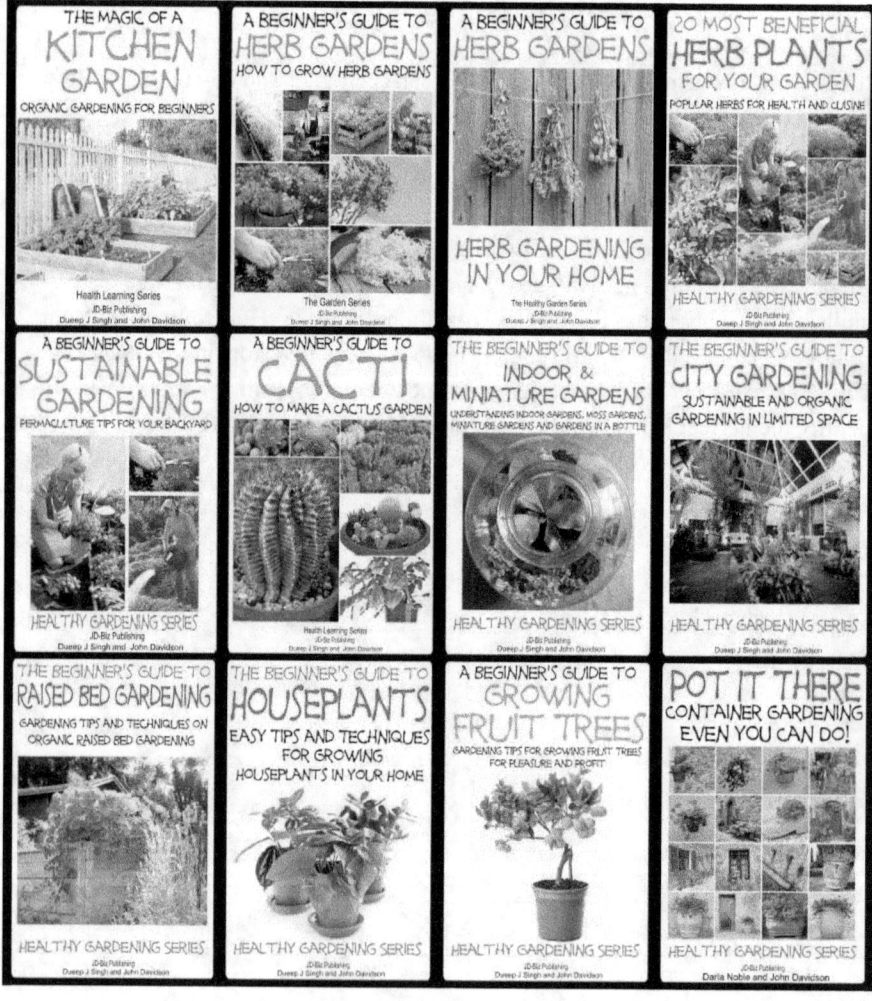

Health Learning Series

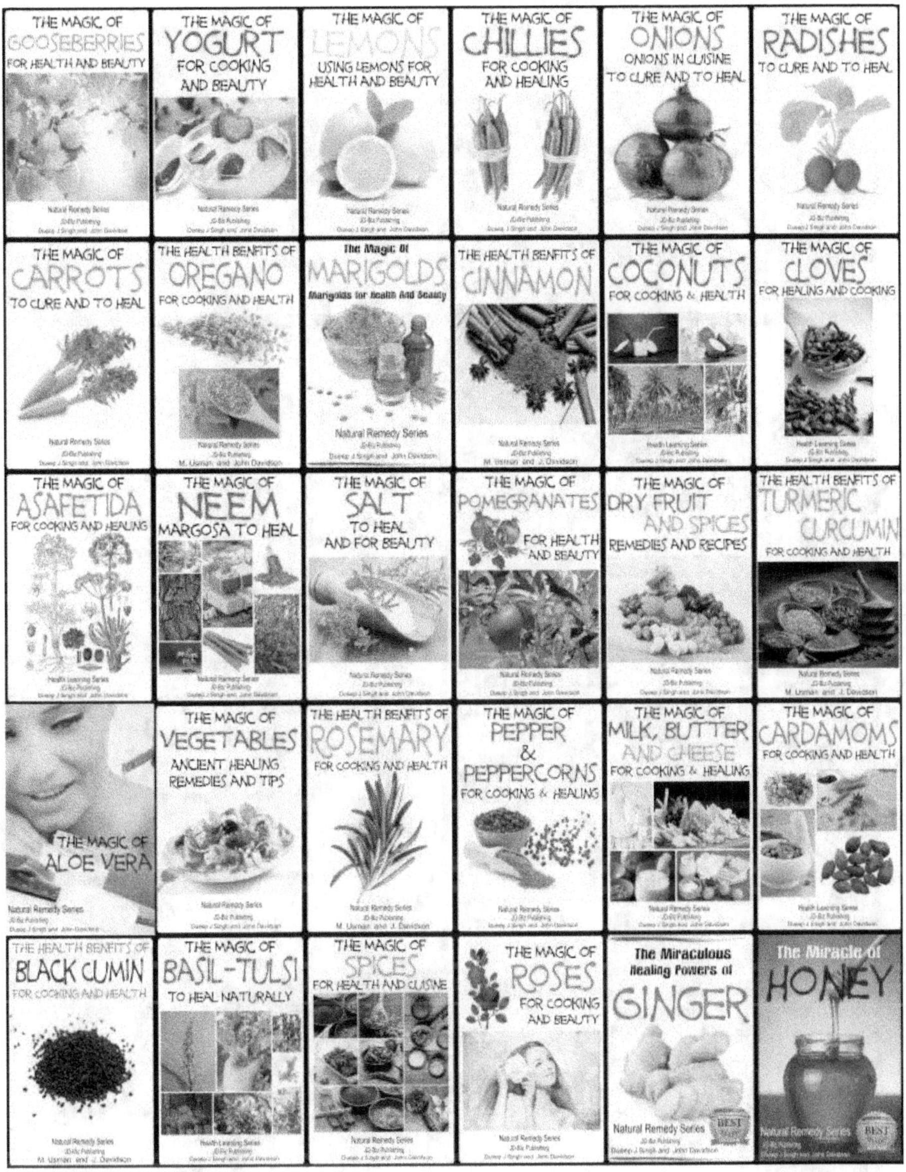

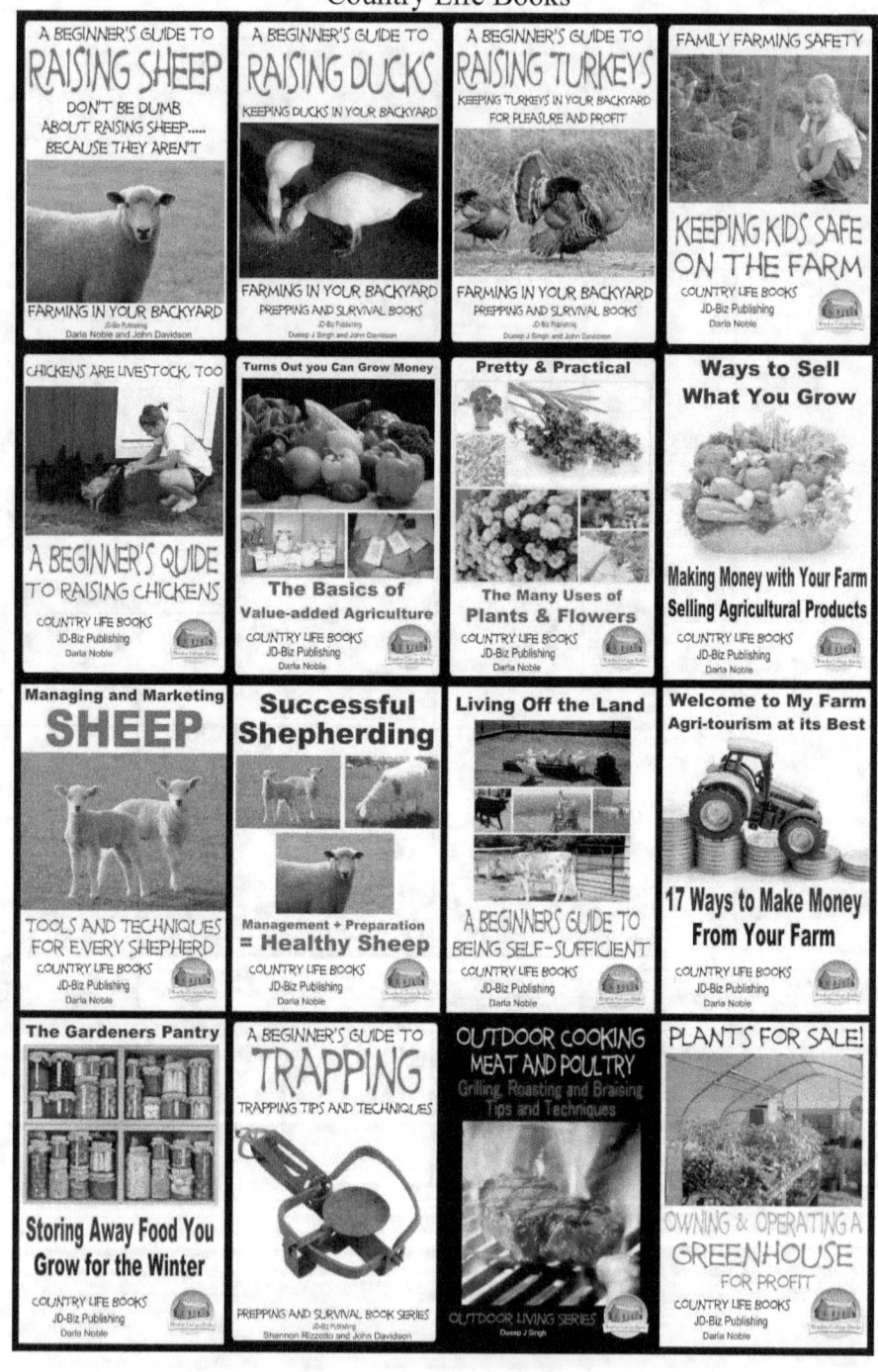

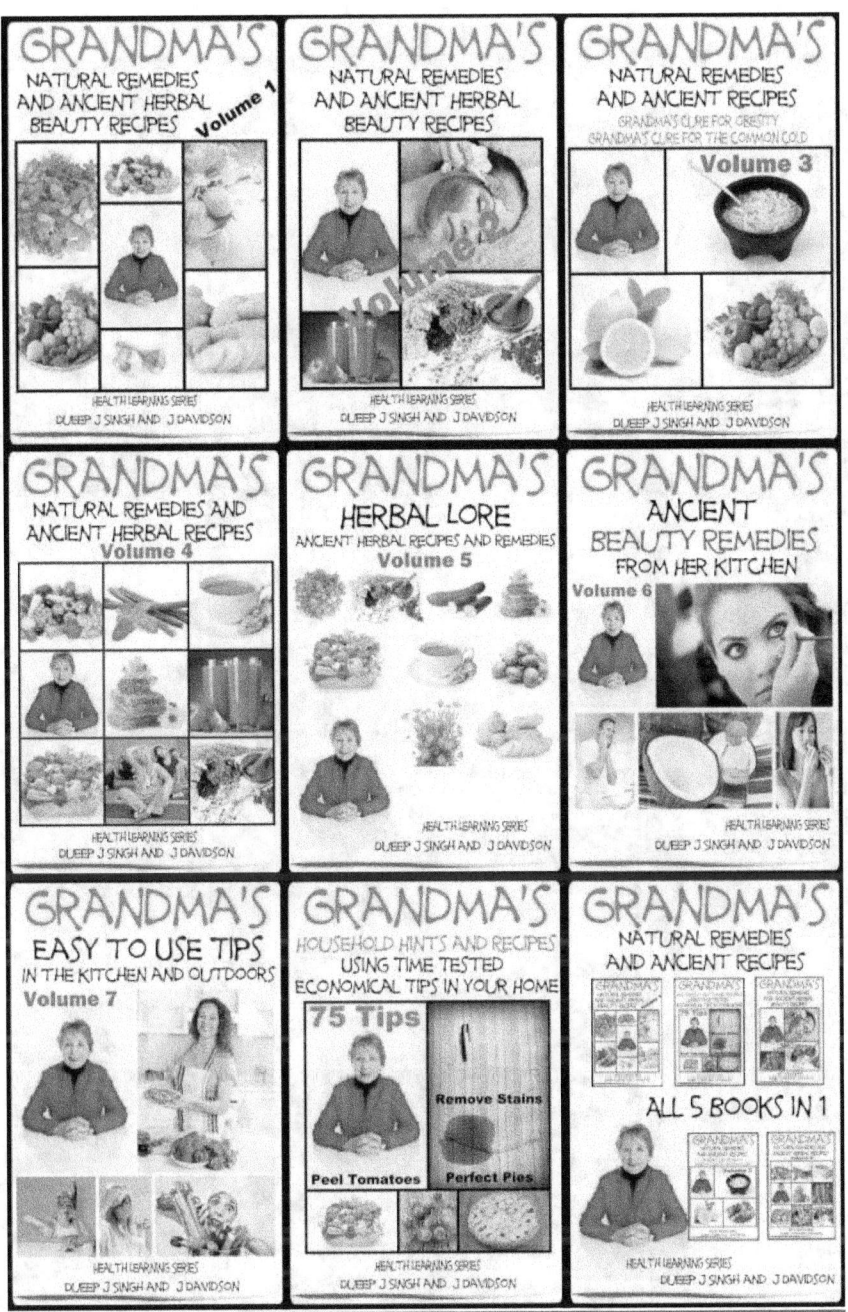

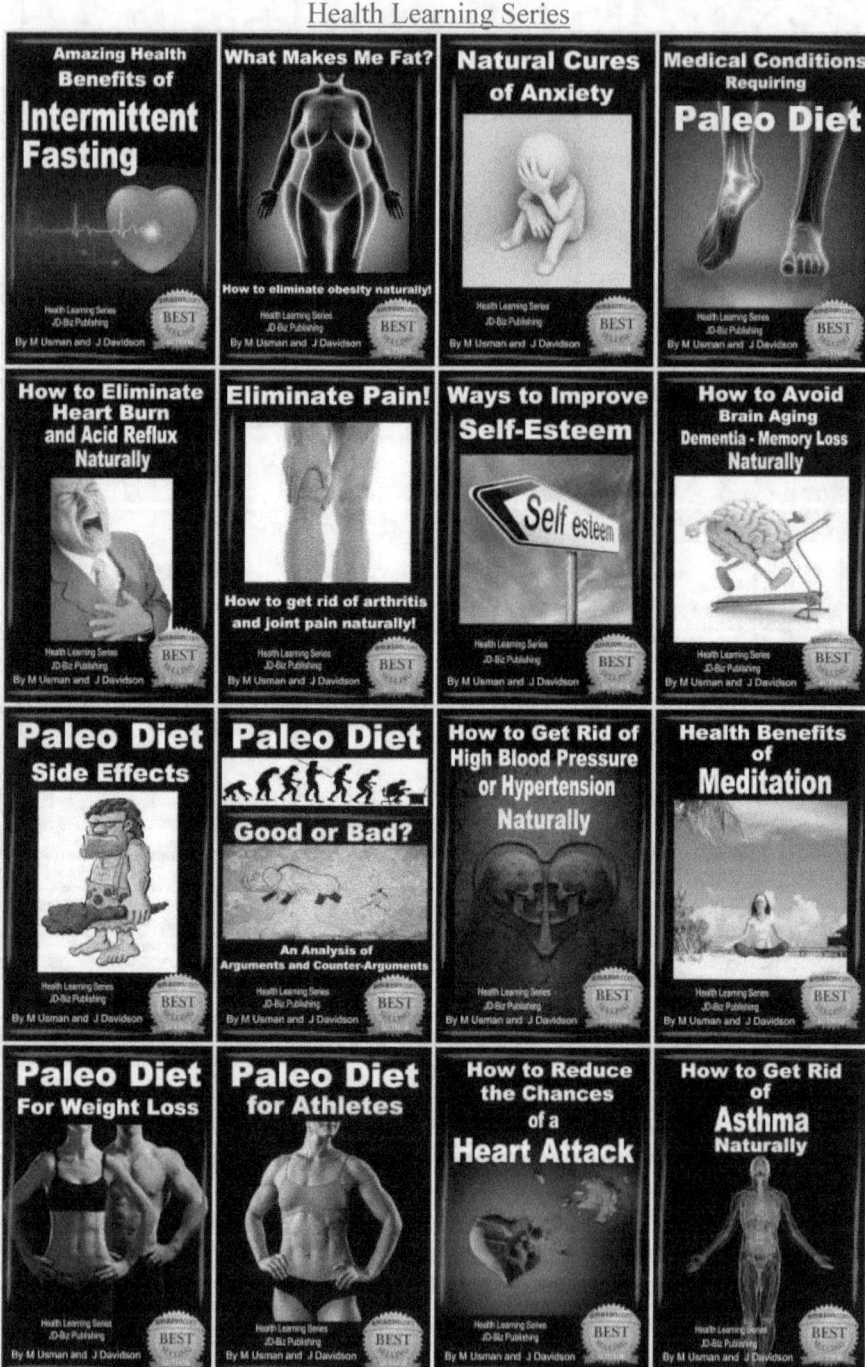

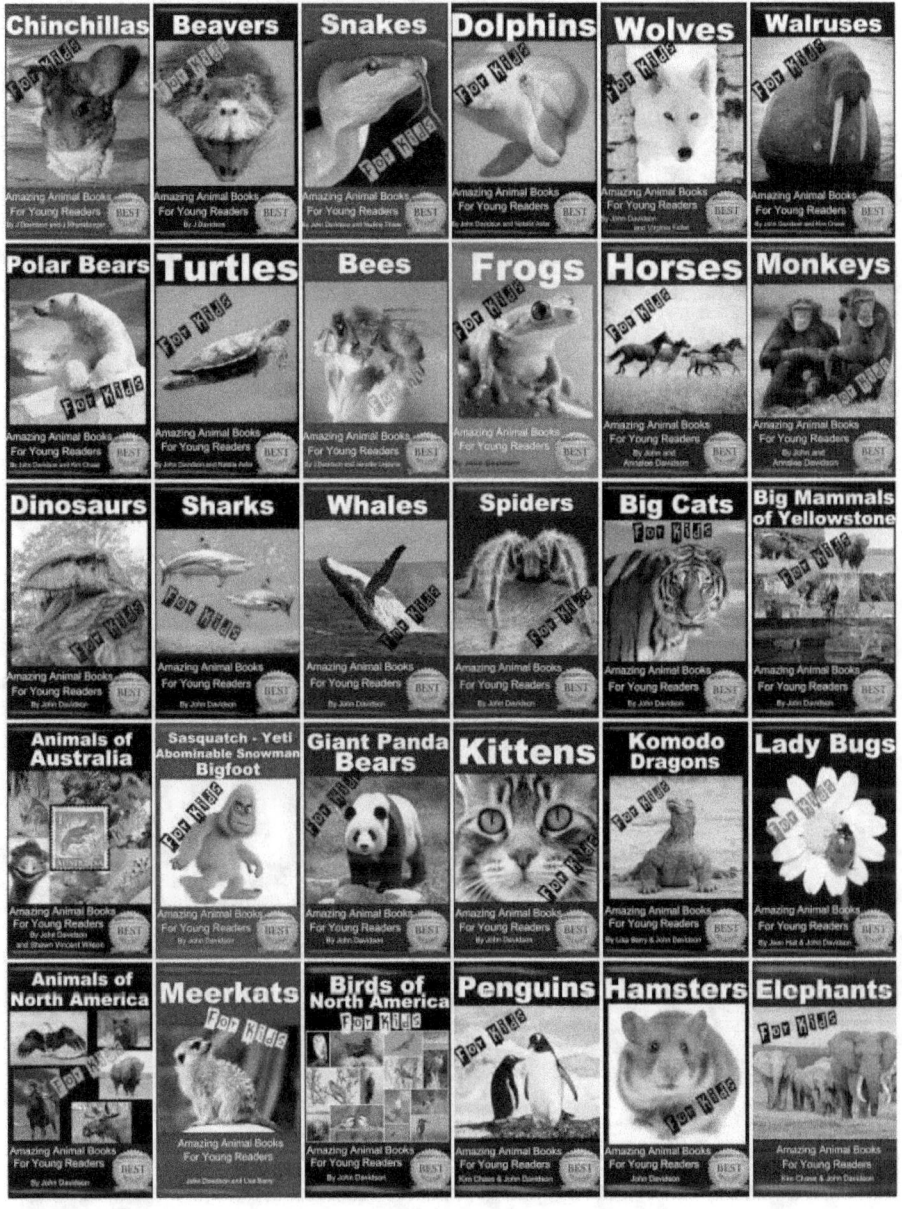

Learn To Draw Series

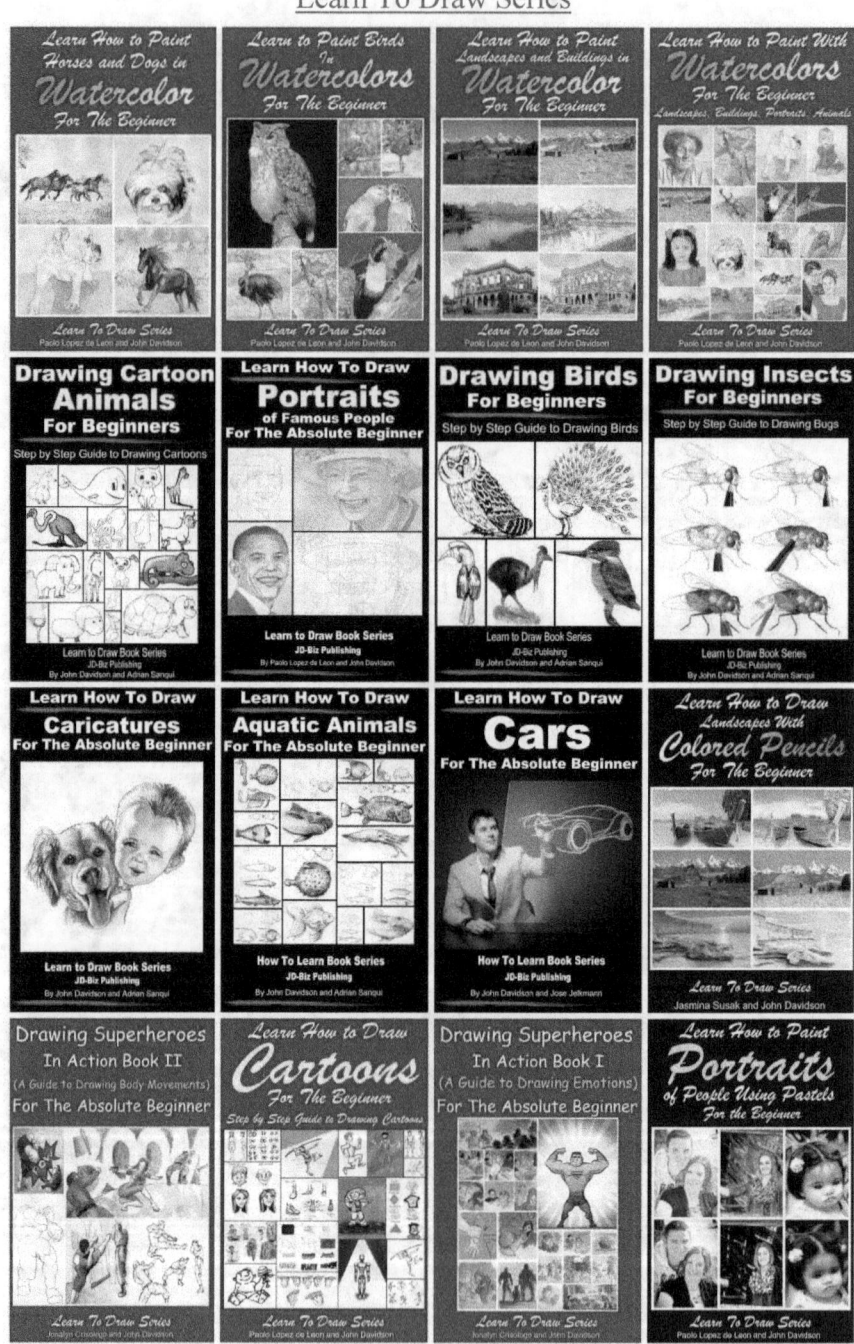

How to Build and Plan Books

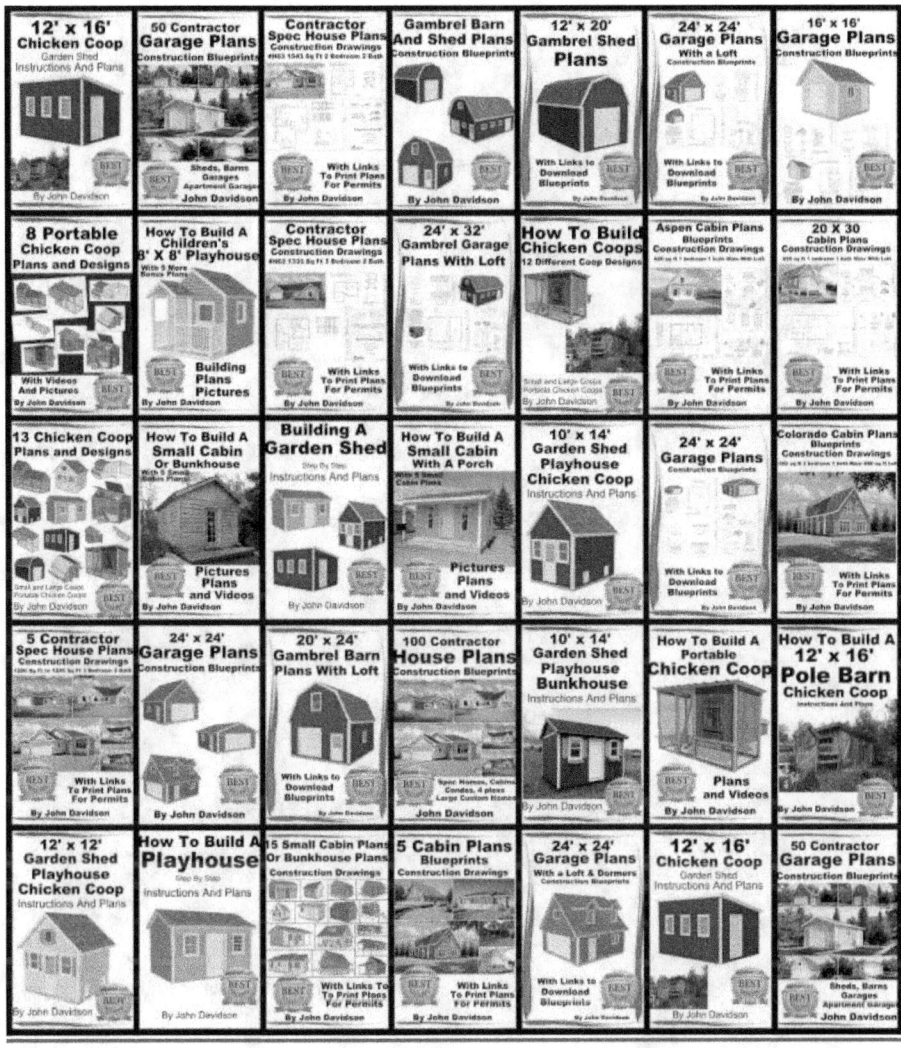

Entrepreneur Book Series

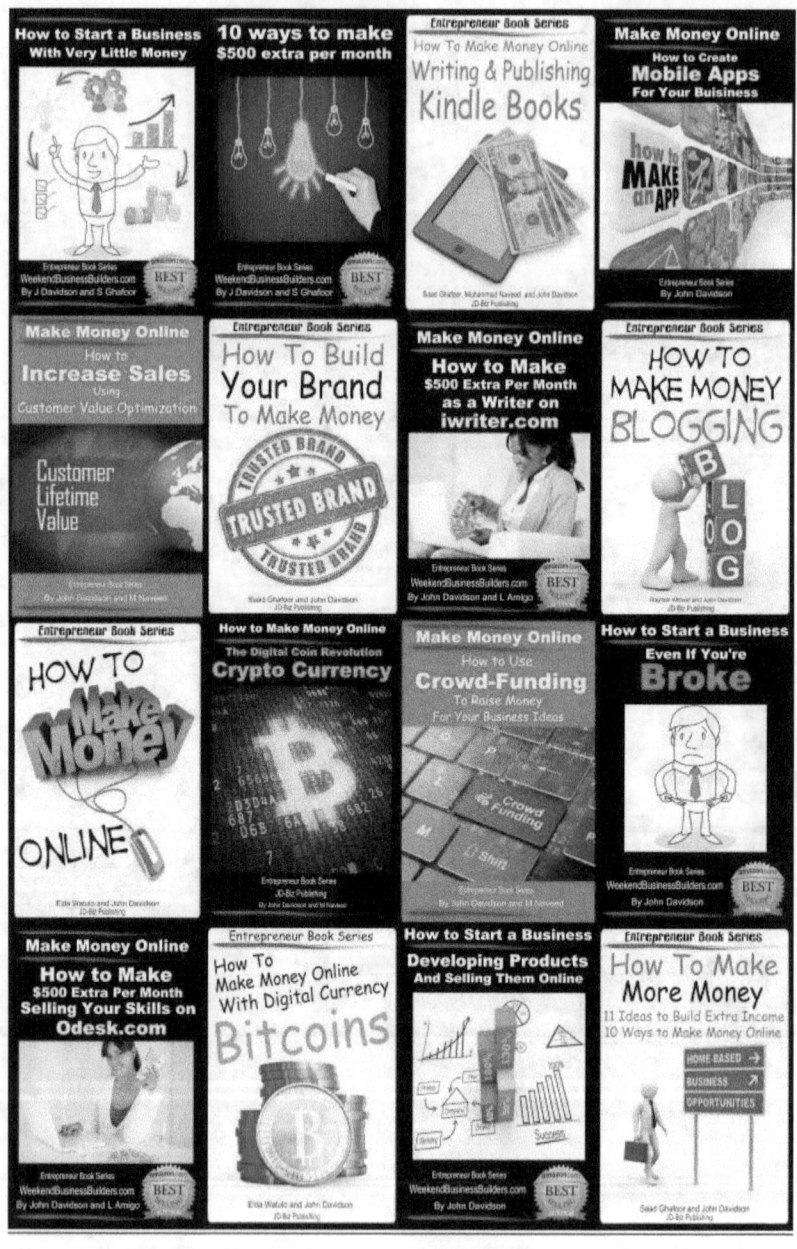

Publisher

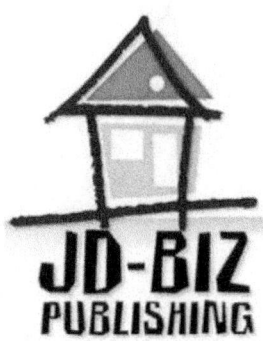

JD-Biz Corp

P O Box 374

Mendon, Utah 84325

http://www.jd-biz.com/

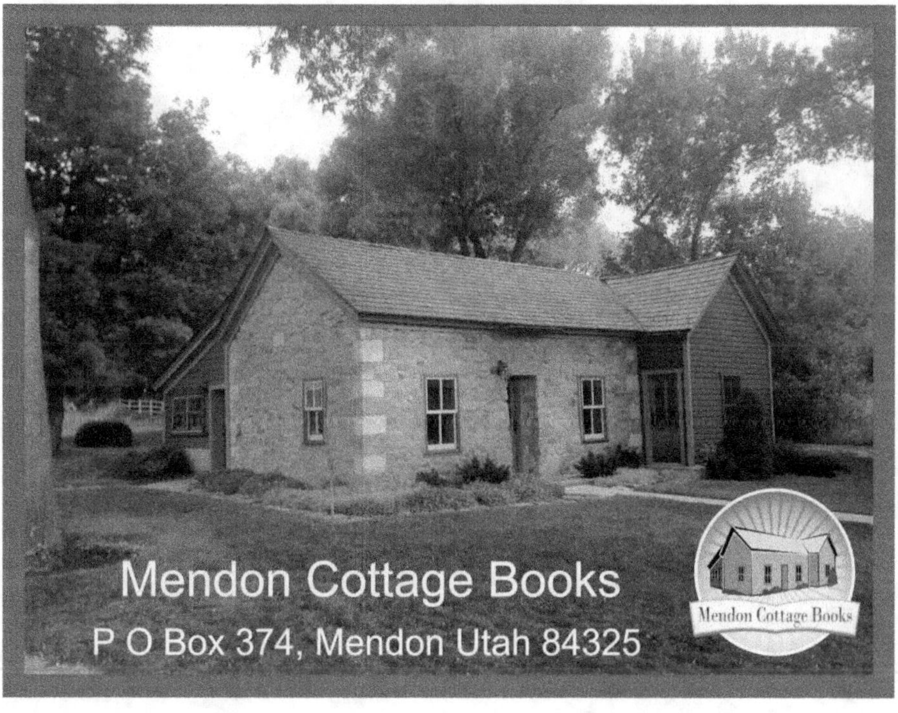

Mendon Cottage Books

P O Box 374, Mendon Utah 84325

www.ingramcontent.com/pod-product-compliance
Lightning Source LLC
Chambersburg PA
CBHW060444290526
45793CB00002B/566